Otherwise, the patient's family has the reality of the situation, that is, what they need to hear, not what they want to hear, have you realized, my brothers and sisters? Is this, and in any case the Prophet said, "Shall I not tell you your wickedness?" They said yes if you want O Messenger of Allah, look at the literature, they say to the Prophet yes if you want, O Messenger of Allah, and he said who descends alone,

began with whom? By the selfish, these said the wickedness of the servants of God, especially the evil of the Companions, he said the one who descends alone, travels and goes and always comes alone, that is, he is unique and not social, he said who descends alone and prevents his support, does not give or help anyone, says God opens for you, someone said Peace be upon you to God, benefactors, and he said to him these do not exist, who you ask about do not exist, did you understand? Someone knocked on the door of the house and said, Peace be upon you, to God, benefactors, and he said to him these do not exist, those you ask about do not exist, the benefactors do not exist, go and knock on another door, and this is true and it is true because it is not one of them, the prophet said who descends alone and prevents his support, that is, he does not give, he does not beat a drop as it is said, his hand is like a rock because of miserliness - God forbid - and keenness and scarcity, God said and souls brought scarcity ⚖, people destroyed incitement and scarcity, the Prophet says and flogs his servant, this goes hand in hand With his descriptions, that is, it is Syndrome as they say, there is no selfish human being who is merciful and loving, this is impossible of course, the selfish is cruel, the selfish is stingy, do not tell me so and so is selfish and he is very generous, this is impossible because the two qualities do not meet, the selfish is very normal to be stingy and it is very natural to be cruel, look at the wise prophet, where are you, Einstein, and you mentioned Moses and Jesus to us and you did not mention Muhammad because you do not know the heritage of Muhammad? And this is not his defect, the shame of Muslims is that they did not inform the world of Muhammad's heritage, they did not do well to show him a good show, it was said a sword and a Qur'an and we brought you slaughter, God willing, Muslims, you have reached the religion of Muhammad, you have reached the religion of the mercy of the worlds with a sword and a Qur'an, they said to people, pay attention and associate between the Qur'an and the sword, the first thing you hear the word Qur'an remember the sword, damn you and this foolish slogan, that is, the logo of a sword and a Qur'an, anyway we do not have to do this, the Prophet said he descends alone and prevents his support And his servant is flogged, Ugh, the companions understood this syndrome, that is, this syndrome, he said, "Didn't I tell you any human beings of that?" Which of this selfish slave, there is still someone who is evil from him, who, O Messenger of Allah? He said those who hate people and people hate them, one of them hates hate, he lives on hatred, so this has to do with my subject, a hated human being and God forbid, he spews hatred, and it is natural to call for hatred so pay attention, now in psychology and science edge psychology they say all negative feelings - of course in the head of hatred and hatred and grudge - would attract to it analogues, hatred can not call tenderness and sympathy - sympathy - and empathy - Empathy - and giving, generosity and cooperation, this is impossible of course, the psychology in which

Hatred that calls for scarcity, exclusivity, hatred, keenness, backbiting, gossip, corruption, seeking reports, prostitution, injustice, tyranny if possible and finally crime, right? I told you that the great Spanish philosopher Ortega y Gasset knew hatred, he said what is hatred? Look what this philosopher said, he said hatred means in the end is killing by force, that is, it is possible, hatred is the readiness of crime, who knows how to hate knows how to kill, so beware, who knows how to really hate knows how to kill, it is normal to kill, especially if he secures the punishment and the circumstances - as I said - and help him, God forbid, we return again to our topic, so whose evil is this? Those who hate people and people hate them, Ugh, I seek refuge in Allah from this characteristic, the Prophet said, "Shall I not tell you any of that?" Yes, if you wish, O Messenger of Allah, those who do not say a stumbling block and do not accept an excuse and do not forgive a sin said, "What is this name?" Hatred, Wilk, if you step on someone on a side, knowing that his father and mother – obviously these are educational matters – taught him this, he brags about himself and claims to be a hero, and we tell him to go and do this with intelligence and darkness and with colonialism and so on, how do you do this with your brothers, your countrymen and your religious people? He says I am a good human being, but do not trample me on a limb, and God who will trample me on a limb I will cut off Dabur and Dabur who gave birth to him, why, my love? Who are you? The Lord of the worlds, people disbelieve in Him and abide by Him, and He blesses you and revives them – there is no god but Him – and opens the door of repentance for them, removes their stumbling blocks, and accepts to forgive them in the last strobe before they die, and

He is the Lord of the worlds, who am I and who are you? Tuck me on my brain and apologize to me and I will tell you God forgive you brother, we are all that wrong, I will not say tuck on my side, but tuck on my brain from above, Abu Dhar – may God be pleased with him – Talahi with Bilal and there was an argument and dispute between them, so he said to him, O son of the black, and the Prophet loved Abu Dhar very much and he used to say tell me Khalili and told me Khalili and singled me out Khalili, the Prophet always said this because he loves him very much, but when he saw this he did not like it, I love you For God and in God, do not the eyes of your devil on you, he said to him the kindness of the saa, that is, the Prophet told him the matter is unbearable, this is the meaning of the tuff of the saa, the Prophet said to him the kindness of the saa, O Abu Dhar that it is not for the son of the white virtue over the son of the black only piety that you are a man in you ignorance, he told him this is one of the characteristics of ignorance, this is not one of the characteristics of monotheism, this is not one of the characteristics of Abdullah, this is not one of the characteristics of faith, how beautiful our religion, what a sweet Islam and God Almighty, I swear By God, how sweet is Islam, oh the loss of young people who are trying to overdo this Islam quickly, they said the Islam of ISIS and the Islam of killing we do not want, and by God, if the whole world became Daesh, I would not have left my religion and I swear by God on this, I swear by God, if all Muslims - all of them from the last - became Daesh and said ISIS is the truth, I would have told you you lied and made a mistake because I know my religion, my religion is not like this and I will not leave my religion, what is my relationship with ISIS and non-ISIS? Do not leave this beauty, do not leave this divine legacy, the world - by God - becomes poor

without Islam and I swear by God on this, without Islam - and God - the world lacks,

this religion is a great extension of life and it was extended thanks to God, do not

judge the great Islam enlightening the mistakes of its children and the madness of its

children and the crimes of its children, do justice - do justice to yourselves and do

justice to the facts - otherwise you are one of the darkest darkness, and we return to

our topic, the Prophet said this is, these - God forbid - the people of hatred, do not

trample on one of them on a party because it does not Forgive, not forgive, and

dismiss? I seek refuge in God, I seek refuge in God, it is one sin with him - one

negligence or a small detail - and brings his enmity forever, the Prophet said these

are the evil of the servants of God, God does not abound in the nation of Muhammad

from them or in human beings from them, I seek refuge in God from them, you see

that the Prophet in his speech gradient up or down? Graded down, worse and worse,

and where was the beginning? Selfishness when he said come down alone, happy

with himself and revolves around himself deified, selfishness is one of the origins of

all evil, self-love and narcissism, the important thing is that we now conclude with the

fourth thing, he said don't I tell you any human being? The what? Is there anyone

more cursed than this too? There is, they said yes, O Messenger of Allah, if you wish,

he said who does not hope for his good and does not believe in his evil, is this the

worst or not the worst? The one who accepted him you are safe unless you step on

him on a limb, but this does not trample him on a limb or on a brain while you are far

from him and yet there is no use and he is cursing you, it is said this heretic who is in the second continent we want to get rid of him, we are in Asia and he is in Australia

but he is a heretic and the son of such and such and we must get rid of him, man I

am in Australia and you are in Asia or in Africa, what is your story with me? The

Prophet said, "Do not hope for his good and does not believe in his evil, may God's

prayers be upon the teacher of good people, the Prophet graduated us and brought

us down lower and lower and lower, that is, the Prophet took us from darkness to a

darker degree, so we stopped seeing, then to a darker degree, then to a very, very,

very dark degree, which is a foul degree and reminds of death, graves, and the

depths of the graves, one of these people said to you, "Do not please his good and

do not believe in his evil, and so is a person if he does not make a covenant with himself and
persevere." With education, discipline and struggle, cleverness is not to

read books and hear words and then review them on people like you, is not so clever,

cleverness in raising yourself, Lord yourself and strive to make yourself better or else

you will lose, you have one life, and all of us, my brothers - God willing - we have

become old, the percentage of young people in us is few, and if we say the average age is
eighty years and this fifty and this forty and this sixty, this means that we - God willing - are
close to death, we We see the other slope of the mountain, I will die and

you will die and he will die and she will die and my neighbor will die and my father

and mother and my teacher and my sheikh and the baker and the drummer and the

plumber and the pharmacist and the doctor and the engineer and the tram driver will

die, everyone will die, he will spend eighty years in this wonderful world, how

wonderful this world is and how wonderful this world is - and God Almighty - when we

take it as a guide to God and a way to God - there is no god but him - and we buy the mole with it, we buy with it forever and buy with it next to God in eternal life and I am

not happier, How beautiful this world is, but we waste these eighty years in gossip,

hatred, hatred, battles, absurdities and sophistry, they are lost from us and there is no second
role, there is no second life, in exams there is a first role and a second role,

right? But in this there is no second role, you missed the opportunity, so be wise and

think a lot, before you send your tongue like a sword and speak and so on, sit in your

house and close the doors on yourself and think a lot about the principles from which

you want to start in driving the vehicle of life, pay attention, the matter is serious, be serious and
do not deceive yourself and do not justify to yourself. So the feelings of

hatred are dangerous in religion, very, very, very dangerous, the Prophet said hatred

is the dream, but I am not saying shaving the hair, but shaving the religion, God

forbid, hatred is abhorrent, but why do we hate? We want to address collective

hatred, of course, which is more dangerous, why do we hate each other? In short,

without dwelling on us, we say that no individual hatred finds its root in the intellectual

or cognitive at all, that is, I cannot hate you and hate me because of the difference in

views on cognitive and scientific issues, impossible This is not the reason, and who

tells you this lies to you and lies to himself, so what? This is not my words, but it is

the words of the geniuses of scientists who began to study the subject, unfortunately

the topic of hatred was not studied accurately as a subject until decades ago, it was

underestimated, but decades ago psychologists and sociologists began to study the

subject of hatred - hatred - and its causes, but before this they did not care much

about it and did not philosophize much about this topic, but now it is different, there is

a book by a very famous scientist and it is anyway from a conference, and this scientist is the editor and her name is Margaret Miller Margaret Miller, the book is

called The Birth of Hatred, which means the birth of hatred, and it is an important

book, this is one of the most important contemporary studies in the philosophy of

hate, and scientists participating in this conference in America are credited with it,

this book is very important, in short, the message of this book says that hatred is not

a simple feeling, but it is a complex feeling, and it is at the end of the analysis a

pathological feeling, no one practices hatred and hates others - even individuals of

course - unless he has a psychological disorder - this man is troubled Psychologically

– or he has internal accusations and suffering that did not reach the disorder –

Disorder – but it is with this poor person, and in the end he is not a psychologically

correct person, the correct psychological does not hate, when you disagree with him

he tells you there is no problem, this is your opinion and this is my opinion and peace

be upon you and it is over, when he sees something you do not have, he says to you, God bless
you, what is the problem with this? He who gave you will give me, this is

God's command, I cannot say otherwise, why am I forcing you to do God? This is

God's action, not yours, who made you rich and made me poor? Is He not the Lord of

the worlds? God said, We divided their livelihood among them, but this one claims

that he is a believer and that he overlooks and he sheds the flames of his hatred on

you and hates him because you are better than him in money or in science or in

beauty or in power or in lineage or in job or in anything, and then he hates you, and I say to you
to be clear in fact this is doubtful in his faith, that is, in the essence of faith

and not in the faith of the tongue as if he says there is no god but God, in essence

Faith is very doubtful, this does not hate the slave, but hates his Lord of course, and I tell you the psychology of atheism – the psychology of atheism, that is, the

psychology of atheism – teaches us and tells us more atheists are not their case that

the evidence of faith did not suffice them, that is, they did not atheist cognitively and

scientifically because the evidence does not convince them, God willing, the

evidence that convinced Aristotle and Plato is unable to convince this great

philosopher who is smarter than Aristotle, but it convinced Al-Ghazali, Ibn Rushd and

Thomas Aquinas Thomas Aquinas, Rene Descartes, Leibniz, Isaac Newton and

Albert Einstein and yet you did not convince him is what God wills, you did not

convince him because he is smarter than them, but atheist psychology says most of

these atheists are not their issue that they do not believe in God but hate God, of

course this is very accurate, they hate God and hate His existence and meeting Him

and that He really exists, do you know why? Because they hate themselves, God

said, they forgot God, and they forgot themselves, and one of them hates himself,

hates his form, hates his lineage, hates his name, hates his destiny, says why am I

so? Why am I not? He hates and therefore is unable in a believing society and in

front of a deceived soul entitled – Title Faith and the motto of faith to say to himself I

really hate God, so I must review my faith from the beginning and see what the

solution is, I must present myself to psychiatrists and psychiatrists, he tells us I hate

you, he says look brother at this hate, look at what he looks like and how he looks,

why is he hateful? He is one of the sweetest people and one of the kindest people

and people love him, he says they are deceived in him and I seek refuge in God from

him and my brother I swear by God that he is such and such, he is poor and then he entered into some of it because he is tired, one of the wise what does he say? Love

blinds us – Blinds us – from mistakes To Default, the Prophet says your love is blind

and deaf, when I love you I don't see any mistake in you, right? The eye of

satisfaction for every defect is blunt, but the eye of indignation shows the equal. He

ceases to see even the virtues that you have, it is clear that you are humble and it is

clear that you are good and it is clear that you are generous and that you are a lover

and the son of respectable and moral people, but he does not see all this, I am angry

with you, so why do you not see him with the eye with which he sees him? He is such

and such and such, this poor person is tired, I tell you - as I said a little while ago -

any poor person who hates and knows hates people and justifies and philosophizes

his hatred is a paralyzed exhilarating, Martin Luther King Jr - the son of course told a very
beautiful phrase, he said what? He said hatred confuses – Confuses – life, and

love is coordinated by Harmonises, hatred confuses life, and love coordinates and

tones it, look at these people, these are the wise men that Einstein talked about,

these people we learn from them and take their language and even take these

quotes of their own because they indicate a deep wisdom distilled from experiences

and readings and from deepening and from many things, they are great men without

a doubt, he said hatred paralyzes – Paralyzes – life, and love releases it, hatred

darkens – makes it dark – life, and love illuminates it, this Look at this hatred to

understand it and to hate hate, so what does Martin Luther King Jr say in another

socket? The martyr, of course, who was killed in the year sixty-eight unjustly and

aggressively, says I have decided to take the path of love, hatred is too heavy to

bear, O peace, he said it is very heavy so I can not carry it, and it is certain that he admires the people who can carry it How do you have the ability – as I said at the

beginning of the sermon – does hatred not delight you? How to carry it and walk with

it? In fact, you do not walk, you are sitting, you are paralyzed as he said, and you

think yourself creative but you are paralyzed, and look at yourself and you will not find a drop of creativity, it is impossible to have any creativity, this is impossible of course, I challenge you to see any person who is hateful and breathes and breathes

hatred and teaches hatred as if he were creative even in anything, I challenge him to be creative, this is not possible, creativity wants freedom and wants to launch and

wants lightness like the lightness of a bird, and this does not He gives her only love,

people must be loved, forgiveness and tolerance, this is it, so one of you may tell me

how to excel, Adnan? And I tell him the first thing is to reduce hatred, what does this

have to do with creativity? This is very important, this is a prerequisite, if you meet all

the conditions and you have hatred that remains paralyzed, remains a sterile personality, we return to our unanswered question, why do we hate each other? Because – as we said – we hate ourselves and hate our destinies and hate those who remind us of what we hate in ourselves, and we do not declare ourselves that we hate this in ourselves, one of us says I am satisfied with the opposite I am very

satisfied with myself, my brother, I - by God - like Diogenes of Sinope, Alexander the

Great son of Philippos came once and stood by the horse on a sunny day in front of

Diogenes and said to him, Diogenes, how are you? How is your news? He is a man

living in a barrel, he said to him, I am in a better situation, and he said to him,

Diogenes, if you were not Diogenes, you would wish you were like whom? Certainly,

he meant to say like Alexander the conqueror of the world, he said to him if I were not

Diogenes, I would wish to be Diogenes, Alexander was annoyed, of course, he

challenged the inner arrogance that he has, which is the arrogance of a great conqueror, he said to him, do you have a request for permission? He said to him, I

have a request, and Alexander rejoiced in this, pay attention to this, so the adults
who have internal tyranny and inferiority complexes and are of power and power, do

you know when they hate you? If, of course, your reason calls because of them – and

hopefully forbid you and I protect you from this, you don't want them – when do they

hate you? If you make them feel dispensed, if you dispense with them, I don't want

your money, I don't want your jobs, I don't want your certificates, I come to advise and

to do good and I don't want anything from you, they hate you so much, why?

Because you make them feel helpless now, they feel strong if you allow them to

humiliate you and enslave you, even if they give you millions they bought you and

enslaved you, when you refuse this with fathers and noses they are very angry with

you, small tyrants as well, such as your manager in the company and your imam in

the mosque, there are - by God - imams tyrants and God forbid, one of them is very

angry with anyone who fixes an issue for him or disagrees with him in opinion or says

something to him, he gets angry and goes crazy, and some of them directly slip into

atonement, a few days ago he sent me One of my loved ones is a video – video – an

engineer by God, and he said to me, look, doctor, is there even atonement in this? I

heard the clip and did not know whether to laugh or cry, by God, these are funny

tears, he said anyone who mocks the clothes of the clergy disbelieves, this is kufr

and then takfr if you do and you do not know, kufr what? What is this stupidity? Kufr

what, man? I mock you and your beard and do not disbelieve, this is empty talk, they

laugh at people and ask people to be really very fearful in front of them and even in front of their clothes, and of course it is interpreted and says this is a year and when

you mocked it you did not mock me, but I - by God - in fact mocked you you frankly, I

did not like your look, not more than this, am I mocking Muhammad? me, and God's

curse is on me to the end of religion and the world if you mock Muhammad peace be

upon him, Muhammad the dust that he walks on over all of our heads, but he wants

to clothe you against your will wrong and say you mean to mock the Messenger of

God Oh heretic and you could not address his mockery until you mocked me, knowing that all
his goal is to cut your tongue off him, they like people to look at them

in a special way, and this is a horrible thing and a hateful thing, the Prophet was not, when
Someone came and cursed Abu Bakr in his face and said to him about you

such and such, knowing that he was a caliph, and someone said to this man I have

disbelieved, Abu Bakr said to him, shut up, there is no one after the Messenger of

Allah, the only Messenger of Allah who if he insults him disbelieves, he said to him even if he
insults me he does not disbelieve, who am I? And today it is not Abu Bakr

al-Siddiq who curses, look and learn, like these one of them says who is Abu Bakr?

He is the friend of the nation and God has said as they are in the cave 🏛, he is the

friend and he is such and such and this man when he cursed him wanted to insult his

prophet is an infidel heretic and beat his neck, and this is a way of understanding and not
stupid, I swear to God this is a way of Satan, what is this jurisprudence? Damn

this jurisprudence, that is, the jurisprudence of these. In any case, we are tall and we

entered into other topics, we come back and say that we - as I told you - hate each

other because of our helplessness, because we remind each other of what bothers

us in ourselves, this intelligence reminds me of my stupidity, and then I get angry and hate him,
because he reminds me that I am stupid, the village preacher who thought

himself Abu Hamid Al-Ghazali or Abu Al-Faraj bin Al-Jawzi because he preached in the village for twenty years when a new preacher came educated and has higher

degrees and a speaker and a speaker and a listener and quick-witted and strong

casual and present argument And strong continuous became very hated and begins

to hunt him, not for the sake of science, exhortation and religion, just because he

underestimated his size in front of people, you as a preacher you were in the eyes of

people a giant, but a real giant came and you reverted a dwarf in the eyes of people,

and this is normal because people compare, he hates him very much and the battle

becomes religious, and this is a lie of course, it is a personal psychological

disturbance, do you understand? I hate this because it reminds me – for example – of my
lineage, they say about him came the prince son of the prince son of such and

such and this is what God wills, these are masters, my brother, and this is a

descendant of the Messenger of Allah, your blessings, our master, and this lineage is

despicable and may even be challenged in his lineage, so this poor man gets very

angry and begins to stab Mr. Sharif, my brother, this is a descendant of the

Messenger of Allah, what is your relationship, man, the shame of this talk, shut up and do not
alert people to the meanness of your origin in this losing battle, but it is

The poor man does and claims to hate him for objective reasons, and the reasons are always
personal, anyway did you understand the message? We come to the

most important part now and the last in the sermon, what matters to us is systemic

hatred, and here one of you may say to me what is the meaning of systemic hatred?

Universal evil, what is it? When you hate a group of people – such as hating a

people, a nation, a sect, a sect, a religious person, or a sect – you don't even have a

personal relationship with them sometimes, what do you think? It is possible that a person belongs to a religion or sect in a country where there is no one of these hated

sect – they are in other countries – and he sees them on television – only – and he

does not see them in reality and does not eat them or sit them and does not have any personal
problem with anyone of them except that he hates them all and wishes to

annihilate them and kill them all, and we used a few days ago to one of these and he says if
they were a billion and a half we would have loved to kill them all from the last of them, Ugh,
What is this capacity for hate? An abnormal ability and a frightening

ability and it is the size of the universe, this is a terrible thing, he wishes to kill a billion and a
half, this is strange brother, this thing is very strange, what is this? What's

going on here? This is what we now want to dismantle quickly, in the last twentieth

century the first to study this case and pay the price, of course, and it is lost in a

scientific and philosophical study for the first time, the Jewish political philosopher

who suffered a kind of suffering from Nazism, of course, Hannah Arendt, Hannah

Arendt has a book called Eichmann in Jerusalem: A Report on the Banality of Evil,

knowing that the word Eichmann is pronounced in German Eichmann, but we

pronounce it in Austria here Eichmann, like Adolf Eichmann, In Jerusalem means in

Jerusalem, A Report on the Banality of Evil means a report of trivial evil, Banality

means ordinary evil or trivial evil, what is trivial evil? Hannah Arendt the persecuted

Jew she and her family and people by studying the case of Adolf Eichmann or Adolf

Eichmann came up with this theory, and of course paid a hard price, cursed by the

Jews and Zionists and accused of being self-hating – a self-hating Jew – and that

she hated her people, and she was not, on the contrary, sympathetic to her people

and the victims, but she liked to understand, she said why did you open fire on me? I

liked to understand, knowing that this is like what is happening now, I a few weeks ago praised Al-Azhar and I know what to say because it did not disbelieve ISIS,

because I know that the weapon used by ISIS to kill me and kill you is takfir, so be

careful, it cannot do this until after it disbelieves in the first, so of course if we use the same weapon - God forbid - what will be our advantage over them? We became like

them, Al-Azhar is balanced, and I even said in the commentary that Al-Azhar is not

ISIS, and Al-Azhar does not belong to the Egyptian regime in a friendly form with

ISIS, on the contrary, ISIS threatens Egypt and the Egyptian regime morning and evening and threatens and says that our way to Jerusalem through Egypt and

through the annihilation of the dreaded Egyptian army, however Al-Azhar - God bless

Al-Azhar - moderate and brave, he told words that may not even be at the whim of

power in Egypt, he said no to atonement, we do not like to disbelieve, criminalize, deny, deny and curse But do not disbelieve, so look at this great philosopher, Hannah

Arendt said to them, "Why did you open fire to me?" Why did you want to assassinate

me? She told them this is a moral assassination, you wanted to destroy my

personality as a political philosopher and as a Jew who loves her religion and people,

even though she was Marxist of course, why did you do this? She said I wanted to

understand and just understanding does not mean forgiveness, I want to understand

the case of Eichmann and the situation of Eichmann and even the situation of many, I

do not want to understand the situation of Eichmann alone, but the situation of an

era, a people, a system and Ism, and we will see what the meaning of Ism, this is an

ideology and doctrine that dominated the world at this time, specifically Germany and

its surroundings, right? And then she said I liked to understand, so when the judge

sentenced Eichmann to death, she was pleased with this and said it deserves and

deserves more than this, but I liked to understand, leave me room to understand, and she gave us her profound experience of understanding in this little pamphlet called

Eichmann in Jerusalem: A Report on the Banality of Evil: Report on petty hate.

What's the story? She said in the Western philosophical intellectual tradition in

general from the days of Plato and Aristotle before Plato – because he is his teacher

– until today it was constantly assumed that all evils go back to one root which is

selfishness, you see how serious selfishness was? This means that the Prophet was

walking in the right way and knew what to say, the selfish man does not hope for

good, the traditional Western philosophical thought has always been like this, she

said until this new state appeared, what is it? The state of Nazism, the Holocaust, the

shames and the disasters of Nazism, why? There has been a refraction in the model

– that is, in the Paradigma in German – here, what is this refraction? Before that man

does evil in general - as we said - because he is selfish, that is, there is a personal

root of evil, I know why I hate you and I know why I antagonize you and I know why I

overwhelm you and hate you, this is known of course, there are reasons, whether

they justify or not, but they remain personal reasons and this is a human thing, she

said you wanted to try Adolf Eichmann to achieve justice, and this will not happen,

why? She said because you are trying Eichmann as a person, the man does not

confess and told you that he does not confess any intention he had when he did what

he did for good or for evil, he said I did not like not to serve Jews and I did not like to

harm them, so what are you? He said I am a bailiff's slave, I am an employee of a

mighty bureaucracy, Germany is a country, and of course they had philosophers,

clerics, churchmen, doctors and others, all of them involved in this, it is not Eichmann who did this alone, he told them I am just a very small cog in a giant bureaucratic machine spinning, I was told to transfer these people and move them, I do not look at them neither as criminals nor as victims, they are just numbers, it is said to transfer ten thousand Jews to Auschwitz Auschwitz and I move them, he issued an order for such and such and he issued an order as he asked me, I had no intention neither in good nor in evil at all, he told them this and he spoke with full confidence, knowing that you can see this in black and white clips on YouTube, there is a part of the Eichmann trial available, and the man speaks calmly, he told them I had no intention neither good nor evil at all, I did not treat them - as I told you - not as Criminals and never as victims, oh, that's a new case we're seeing for the first time, isn't it? Hannah Arendt says – it is quite a misfortune and I completely agree with it – from the old ironic tradition to almost today and until before Nazism thought was considered a mirror in which the individual tries to see himself, there is an internal dialogue and you know Socrates' way of dialogue, there is dialogue in the sense that I ask myself

about my motives, about my goals and objectives, about my justifications, why am I doing this? What do I want from this? Is this justified or unjustified? Is this justification given to me in the form of an order justified or unjustified? Is that enough to be a justification? In the sense that the individual should have fought a grueling and exhausting battle in making moral judgments on himself and others, but Nazism forbade all this, this is a thing of the past, in the sense of what? In the sense that it referred the people, referred people, and referred individuals to just machines that only program, just as a robot is programmed to kill, when any person sees a certain attribute killing him, for example, can this robot be tried? I have now simplified for you Arendt theory of trivial evil - The Banality of Evil - or the habitual evil and the banality

of evil, evil has become something that does not provoke any feelings, do and burn

thousands of people and tens of thousands and even millions of people without

blinking an eyelid, without wondering once about the morality of this act or the

suffering of these victims because they are not victims with you, this is normal for you

and you do this while you are comfortable and eat and drink and do not disgust or

vomit, may God have mercy on our teacher Al-Missiri He once said I met one of

them, and he said to me, "I am going to an important journey, Abdel Wahab, will you

come with me?" I told him where? He said I will go to meet Robert Oppenheimer, he

is the father of the atomic bomb project, and he said I told him, of course, this is a

historic opportunity because I will meet Oppenheimer, he is one of the greatest

physicists in the world, he is the father of the atomic bomb project, he said I said I go

and I went to him, and of course Oppenheimer is not only a scientist, but he is a great

philosopher and he was deep in the most extreme Eastern religions and he read and

cites the Upanishads, this man was deep and he was a Jewish person and one of the

The victims of Nazism in America, El-Messiri – may God have mercy on him – said I

took advantage of the opportunity and I told him, Professor Oppenheimer, I want to

ask you a simple question, and he said to him, go ahead, he told him when this bomb

was detonated and what happened, what was your reaction? The man was very

moved by the question and said, "Do you know what my reaction was?" Exactly as it

is, I vomited, Oppenheimer vomited because he is a noble person, he has a deep

humanity, this thing I will not say is evil but it is something ugly and something disgusting and disgusting, man ended with equations and science and philosophy and objective knowledge until his fellow man is killed in this way, hundreds of thousands are burned in an instant, how do we do this? He said I caused this and then I vomited, and of course this man – as you know – was tried and almost spent his entire last life in semi-house arrest, isolated hated because he leaked secrets to the Soviet Union, he said this is not true and then our enemy must have a bomb program in order to make mutual deterrence otherwise we are fools, we Americans will become fools and we will slaughter the world in this way, and this should not, we will give the Soviets atheists this secret in order to restrain us, and this is noble, do you support it? I support him, do you support this betrayal? I support it, this betrayal is excellent because it is for the benefit of humanity, the great Oppenheimer now reminds us of Montesquieu, the owner of the spirit of the laws when he said if I discover something that serves my country France and harms the world and I can offer it to my country I will not offer it, the interest of the world should take precedence over my country, France will destroy the world in the end or will hurt the world, do you understand? I'm sure you've become shocked, you're going to say Ugh, such mentalities – Montesquieu and Robert Oppenheimer – with this logic and with these quotes when we put them on some of the actions of Muslims today we will lose the whole battle, and this is true of course, you will be outside the issue and no one will respect you or anyone who respects your religion, anyone respects, right? You must responsibly, seriously and honestly, reconstruct an Islamic discourse that is like this and even surpasses it, do you understand? This is it, take care of humanity and make the general always your choice, Islam is the religion of the worlds and God is the Lord of the worlds. We go back again, anyway, what did Hannah Arendt say? She said this man – as I said – became like a machine that programmed and then lost his humanity, she said for the first time humanity is witnessing crimes that people do not do, so who is doing them? She said it is done by denials, of course anyone like Adolf Eichmann and does everything he did is a denial, and of course there are people who are much worse than him of course and this is known, but he did everything he did and said he did not bat an eyelid and I did not wonder and I had no intention of good or in evil, so you are a nobody, you are not the man the heavenly books told us about, you are not the man about whom Laozi or Confucius or the enlightened Buddha told us Or Socrates or Plato or Aristotle, that's impossible of course, you're something completely different, it's of course Nothing, you're nothing, you're just a nobody, so Hannah Arendt said to them – how wonderful this philosopher is and how wonderful this book is, and God how wonderful my brother, this is a very wonderful person – you want to achieve justice by trying someone, and that person does not exist If you want to be judged, you must try the ISM, do you know what ISM is? The suffix which means ideology or doctrine like Marxism, Darwinism and Capitalism and so on, she told them to judge the ism, that is, judge the ideology, judge the era, judge the era, judge the era, judge the general framework, don't judge people, this is difficult because people don't exist, she said this is a scary case for the first time we see it, this is what I call the banality of evil, but the word triviality does not mean triviality, which means the existence of something trivial, but it means ordinary, that man does evil as if breathing or It's like drinking cold water, this is not a trait in man,

man doesn't do this, even the great barbarians and Mongols – like Genghis Khan –

and Tatars like them don't do this, speaking of barbarians there is now a very famous

novel by Ji. M. J. M. Coetzee South African name waiting for the barbarians, and it

seems that the name of this South African novel is taken from the name of a poem by

an Egyptian poet Alexandrian origins Greek Constantin Cavafy, known as

Constantine Cavafy, Cavafy has a poem you can find on the net - Net - because it

exists in many sites for Arabic poetry and world poetry, this poem is called waiting for

the barbarians, and it is a simple one-page poem, talking about the parish and that

the king takes his adornment and gift in order to They are waiting for a delegation of

barbarians and they are always their enemies, these are enemies who always

threaten the state on its borders and can assassinate it at home, read of course A

Study of History by Arnold Toynbee to know how this barbaric aggression explains

the destruction of civilizations and nations, which is a well-known story in the philosophy of
history, so these are the barbarians, at the end of the poem what does

Constantine Cavafy say? Say what to me I see the fields have been desolate? Why

do people all go back to their homes or homes and are looming over them, what

happened? The whole Samer broke up without anything happening, what happened?

Listen to this well, he says some soldiers came from the border and told that there

are no barbarians anymore because they will not come to us, and this delegation –

Delegation – of theirs will not come, so go and leave, but the people broke up and

they are sad, although the barbarians represent an imminent danger, and the best thing that happened is that they disappeared and evaporated, and yet the people are

sad and the king is sad and the courtiers and the lining and even everyone is blinded,

because there are no barbarians, you see what happened? This poem in the ninth

century, in the last decade of the nineteenth century, was written by Constantin

Cavafy, the Alexandrian Greek, the important thing is that he finally said in order to

conclude the poem: Now? Without the barbarians, what would happen to us? These

barbarians were a solution. I think this conclusion to this very suggestive and very

deep poem can put the finger on a possible explanation of the state of systemic

hatred, how can you hate an entire nation, an entire people, an entire sect, or a cam

sect even though you have nothing to do with them and you have never seen them

and there is nothing personal, do you know why? Employing a cursed politician, and

this happens whenever I play politics or whenever religion plays politics or wants to

play politics, this is my absolute conviction and I will not abandon it, knowing that this

does not mean that there is no political game, there is a political game in the Middle

East, but what I have been demanding for years and I am still demanding is to play

politics with politics, they exalted the sacred religion, they exalted the religion of the Lord of the
worlds and the religion of all people from employing it, integrating it,

polluting it and desecrating politics with its endless defilement, isn't it Also? Then

politicians are free by God, and of course countries have options and they have

cycles, and then they are free, all politicians have to play politics as they want and

openly without any problem, but keep religion away and exalt religion, knowing that

this is happening to everyone without exception, I do not exclude anyone, do not tell

me I exclude Shiites or others, everyone applies to this, they all play with religion politics and I swear to God on this enough, enough of this play with religion, make

religion away, as I do, for example, I do not try to use religion in politics, and I do not

want to do this at all so that I am not cursed in this world and the hereafter, do this

and play politics away, but unfortunately politics and the management of states and

the management of herds - Herds - require this, humans are treated like herds of

power always, these herds how are they managed and how they walk - walking

asleep - and how they enchant and attract? Do you know how this always happens?

With the danger that looms at her, she is told there are barbarians, if you keep silent

and you are not behind us and do not support us in all our massacres they will eat

you and slaughter you and they will not make you exist, the barbarians will end your

life, right? Before the collapse of the Soviet Union in the late nineties – in the early

last decade – what existed? There was the red danger, that is, the Soviet Union and

communism, it ended – thank God – with cardiac arrest of course, and the Berlin Wall

was an icon – an icon – ending with cardiac arrest, what did the West do here? He

can't live without barbarians, can he? They baptized new people as barbarians, who

are they? Unfortunately, this was of course in Spain – specifically Barcelona – and

the man who was speaking on behalf of NATO – NATO – said the red danger is over

and this will not work, in order to complete our march we need another danger to fear

and so on, he said there is the green danger, knowing that we heard this on

television, that is, this is not secret information, this talk came on television –

television – but the Islamic nation did not understand anything, and from that day I

exploded in my head a great awareness and I was then in Al-Hidaya Mosque and I said watch out, Muslim scholars, leaders and thinkers, watch out, there is a great evil

that is meant for us, we now have to reprogram ourselves and program our speech

so that we do not help ourselves and our religion, pay attention to this, since these

days I have been demanding an excellent version that is humane, merciful and

civilized of religion, and I knew that every barbaric and barbaric and violent version

will facilitate the enforcement of the conspiracy in us and I swear to God on this, so

from the first day I was against bin Laden and against al-Qaeda And I said the same

interpretation, and my words to this day are sincere, God willing, and everything that is being
confirmed by - by God - follow the example of the shell with the shell, but there is no hearing but
a few, there is no sane but a few, people do not reason and do
not understand and then laugh at them, we are today the barbarians of the West, Constantine
Cavafy said:

العالم العظيم عدنان ابراهيم